# Vegan Intermittent Fasting
## Lose Weight, Gain Mental Clarity and Change Your Life

Katie Maria

# Table of Contents

# Chapter One - Intermittent Fasting Explained

*Introduction and History*

In simple terms, intermittent fasting is an eating schedule in which you control the times you do and do not eat during a 24-hour period. Rather than labeling certain foods as good and others as dangerous, intermittent fasting redirects the focus from *what* you consume to *when* you consume it. This consumption period is known as your 'eating window', a set period of time in which you consolidate your total daily calories. The time period outside of this window is when you are fasting, in other words, you abstain from any and all calories. By placing the restriction solely on the time of day you eat rather than on the types of foods you put into your body, intermittent fasting complements a wide variety of lifestyles, including veganism.

While intermittent fasting has only recently become a hot topic in the media, fasting itself can be traced back to the hunter and gatherer societies thousands of years ago. In those earlier times, fasting was more so a way of survival rather than an intentional practice, but nevertheless, it existed. In the decades and centuries that followed, the human species evolved, and so did the practice of fasting. As the hunting and gathering lifestyle became a thing of the past, fasting moved forward with the times and continued to find its way into our more advanced society. Some newer examples of fasting include religious, spiritual, cultural, and scientific settings such as rituals, protests, and medical research.

Religious reasons for fasting are vast and varied, and people have been engaging in such practices all around the world for decades. Christians use fasting as a challenge in order to grow closer to God during the season of Lent, which may even include fasting from activities such as shopping and playing video games. In Islam, it is common to fast during the Islamic holy month of Ramadan as a way to practice resisting goodness. In the Jewish community, fasting on the Jewish holy day of Yom Kippur is a spiritual exercise, based on the belief that depriving yourself of food is beneficial for spiritual growth. These are just examples of some of the many religious practices that exist in our society today, plus a little insight into how they may be tied to culture and spirituality.

In today's world, fasting remains a common practice in both religious practices and other settings mentioned above, but perhaps the most prominent discussion now revolves around the positive effects that fasting can have on the body. This is where 'intermittent' fasting comes into play, a concept first introduced by Martin Berkhan in 2006 which led to a huge shift in the fitness industry. What makes this shift so interesting is that the fundamental principles of intermittent fasting seem to contradict many former beliefs surrounding meal times and meal frequency. For example, 'breakfast is the most important meal of the day' was replaced with 'skip breakfast' and 'eat six small meals every 2 to 3 hours' was swapped with 'eat 2 to 3 large meals in an 8-hour window'. Almost overnight, people seemed to ditch their deep-rooted set of beliefs in favor of this alternative way of thinking. The big question then becomes why.

Despite the seemingly contradictory principles at the foundation of intermittent fasting, the results that people were physically seeing and mentally feeling were far too promising to be ignored. This is when intermittent fasting really started to gain traction, both within the fitness world and beyond. As this new lifestyle spread across the fitness industry and made its way into the news, everyone wanted to understand how this phenomenon actually worked. At the time, intermittent fasting was still a relatively new concept, and there wasn't much information to support the practice, but that's less so the case today. Over the past ten years, a number of studies have been carried out on many different aspects of the lifestyle, and the results are overall favorable. While there is still a great deal of misinformation and uncertainty surrounding intermittent fasting, there seems to be enough evidence to suggest that the benefits outweigh the drawbacks.

Today, intermittent fasting is a way of life for a diverse group of individuals all across the world. The attention that this eating pattern has received from the media and various other outlets in such a short amount of time is truly astonishing. Furthermore, now that some of the fundamental principles underlying intermittent fasting have become backed by credible research studies and reliable scientific sources, doctors and other health professionals are even recommending this way of eating to treat a variety of medical conditions, and patients are reporting incredible results. What makes intermittent fasting so widespread is the fact that it is simple to follow and inclusive of all types of people, no matter their background or prior dietary regimen. By the looks of it, this is just the beginning for the intermittent fasting community, as it seems like the lifestyle is here to stay.

*How It Works*

Cycling in and out of a fasted and not fasted state allows you to control certain functions within your body to make them work better for you. When you consume calories, some of that energy will be stored as glycogen in your liver. After 10 to 12 hours, those glycogen reserves will be nearly depleted, causing the fat cells in your body to release fats into the bloodstream. These fat cells will quickly find their way into your liver, where they are converted into energy. This new form of energy can then be used by your body and brain, so you are essentially burning fat cells to survive. In sum, by eating normally during so-called eating windows and abstaining from calories during periods of fasting, you can turn your body's cellular and metabolic processes into a fat burning machine.

Another term that is often used in connection with intermittent fasting is ketosis. This is a state in which ketones, chemicals released during the body's fat burning process, trigger the release of a neurotransmitter called BDNF, brain-derived neurotrophic factor. This molecule is responsible for building and strengthening both neurons and neural connections in the brain regions that control learning and memory. There is research to suggest that eating a high-fat, low-carb diet can encourage ketone production as well, which is how the ketogenic diet came to be. However, when you compare the ketogenic diet to intermittent fasting, the latter is far more effective for increasing ketone levels. This is why researchers believe that ketosis triggered by fasting could be the key to a longer life and optimal overall health.

Studies show that 16 hours is the bare minimum amount of time that your body must fast in order for these positive benefits to kick in, which is why the 16:8 Method is so common in the intermittent fasting community. This method was popularized by the founder himself, Martin Berkhan, and is an eating pattern in which you fast for 16 hours with an 8-hour eating window, often centered around weight training. Most people who are getting into intermittent fasting for the first time will start with this method, which is sometimes referred to as The Leangains Method in the fitness world. From here, some may work their way up to an 18- or 20-hour fast with a 6- to 4- hour eating window, respectively.

Beyond the bare minimum of 16 hours, it seems that there may actually be exponential benefits with each additional hour that the body remains in a fasted state. More specifically, fasts closer to 16 hours affect body composition while fasts beyond this 16-hour marker reap the benefits of cellular rejuvenation. In other words, something called autophagy occurs, which is the body's natural recycling process of cells. This involves repairing old and damaged cells within the body, a sort of detox process in which old cells get eaten up by newer ones and are then consolidated into more powerful and efficient cells. Results of cellular rejuvenation include, but are not limited to, glowing skin, a longer life, and an improvement in all kinds of organ functions within the body.

*Different Types of Fasting*

The fundamental principles of intermittent fasting remain the same no matter how you choose to look at them, but there are many different ways that you can incorporate these principles into your current lifestyle. Depending on your prior experience with fasting, your day to day schedule, your exercise regimen, and so forth, you may be drawn to one type of fasting over another. These methods vary in their duration of the fasting period and eating window, the calorie allowances while fasting, the frequency of the fasts, and more. There is no right or wrong; it's all about what is going to work best for your lifestyle and help you achieve your goals.

The 16:8 Method -

> The most basic type of intermittent fasting, and the type that is recommended for beginners, involves fasting for 16 hours with an 8-hour eating window. This type of fasting is a form of 'time restricted feeding' since all your daily calories must be consumed within the restricted time of 8 hours. Since the average person naturally fasts for 8 to 12 hours overnight, extending the fasting period to 16 hours usually just means skipping breakfast and late-night snacks. These small adjustments help ease the transition into fasting and is one the reasons that the 16:8 Method is so popular among beginners. Other variations of this method include the 18:6 Method and the 20:4 Method, whereby you fast for 18 to 20 hours with a 6 to 4-hour eating window, respectively.

Alternate Day Fasting -

A more extreme alternative to time-restricted feeding is Alternate Day Fasting, a method in which you eat normally for one whole day and fast for the entire following day. Then you continue alternating between these eating days and fasting days, which is where this method gets its name. The eating days are fairly self-explanatory, but the fasting days leave a bit of room for decision making. Some people choose to abstain from all food on fasting days, consuming only water and other liquids, while others choose to consume up to 600 calories on these so-called fasting days. This latter option is referred to as fasting-mimicking, a type of method which some studies suggest may have a few added benefits of its own.

The 5:2 Diet -

Similar to Alternate Day Fasting, the 5:2 Diet involves eating normally five days out of the week and fasting on the remaining two days per week. These periods of fasting can either be broken up into two 24-hour fasts or one 48-hour fast. This type of fasting is also known as the Fast Diet and was popularized by British journalist Michael Mosley. Again, this diet lets you choose between abstaining from all calories during your fasting periods or entering a fasting-mimicking state, whereby you consume up to 600 calories. The important thing is not to compensate for these fasting periods by consuming more calories on your eating days, as this may lead to weight gain and other unfavorable results.

Eat-Stop-Eat -

The Eat-Stop-Eat style of fasting is normally done once or twice during a given week and involves a 24-hour fast in which you don't consume any calories. One of the most popular ways to incorporate this fast is to abstain from eating between dinner one day and dinner the following day. Of course, you can also choose to fast from breakfast to breakfast, or lunch to lunch. In contrast to Alternate Day Fasting and the 5:2 Diet, this type of eating schedule does not include the option to enter a fasting-mimicking state since the goal is to put your body into ketosis more quickly.

The Warrior Diet -

Popularized by fitness expert Ori Hofmekler, the Warrior Diet is a different type of fasting method in which you fast during the daytime and eat a large meal right before bedtime. The daytime fast still allows you to consume small amounts of raw fruits and vegetables, as well as calorie-free liquids, but most of your calories should be saved for the nighttime feast. This variation of intermittent fasting does recommend that you base your large meal around paleo-friendly foods such as eggs and grass-fed meats, so it may not be the most suitable for vegans. If you do want to attempt this diet as a vegan, a combination of healthy oils, nuts and seeds, and vegetables is your best bet.

Hunger-Centered Fasting -

The Hunger-Centered method of fasting is less popular than other types because it involves truly listening to your body and is really open to interpretation. The basic idea is that you eat when you are hungry, and you don't eat when you are not hungry. It sounds simple, but in today's society where food is always in a large abundance, our hunger cues are completely thrown out of whack, and it can be difficult to tune into the experience of true hunger. Therefore, this type of fasting may work best under the supervision of a healthcare professional who can help guide through your fasts, at least in the beginning.

No matter which of these fasting methods, if any, you choose to implement in your daily life, keep in mind that your diet still needs to consist of healthy, high-quality foods. Abiding by an eating schedule is not the same as swallowing a magic pill, and you will most likely feel crappy if you're eating junk outside of your fasting periods. Also consider whether intermittent fasting is the right choice for you, depending on whether or not it will help you achieve the goals you have set out for yourself. This lifestyle is certainly not for everyone, and while it can be beneficial for some, it may be detrimental for others.

# Chapter Two - Pros and Cons of Intermittent Fasting

*Health Benefits*

The popularity of intermittent fasting is in large part a direct result of the incredible health benefits experienced by the many individuals who have already embraced the lifestyle. While some of these positive health effects are neither understood nor backed by science just yet, the results don't lie. One theory suggests that periodic food deprivation serves as a sort of preconditioning stress, thereby making the human body more equipped to resist bigger stressors in the future. This would make a lot of sense based on the relationship we already know to be true between stress and health, but again, it is not yet accepted as fact. Nonetheless, there are still a number of physical and mental benefits that can be discussed in relation to intermittent fasting, even without having the in-depth scientific explanations to support them.

Preserve Muscle Mass While Losing Fat -

Intermittent fasting is supposedly far more effective at preserving muscle mass during weight loss than any form of deliberate calorie restriction. While fasting may still result in a calorie deficit and therefore lead to weight loss, this occurs more naturally since the focus has been shifted away from the restriction of calories. Further, what makes this way of eating a great method to preserve muscle is the fact that fasting improves insulin sensitivity, which is basically a measure of how responsive your cells are to the hormone insulin. Since insulin sensitivity encourages muscle glycogen synthesis while insulin resistance promotes fat storage, improving insulin sensitivity is highly favorable and is especially beneficial for individuals with type 2 diabetes.

Reduce the Risk of Diabetes -

Diabetes is a condition whereby your body can't produce insulin or is unable to use the hormone efficiently. As a result, your blood sugar ends up being much too high. Since fasting improves insulin sensitivity and regulates your blood sugar levels more effectively, studies suggest that adopting this lifestyle can reduce your risk of diabetes and also reverse type 2 diabetes in those already diagnosed with the disease. While it is still too soon for health professionals to recommend intermittent fasting as a scientifically sound treatment for diabetes, this could change in the near future.

Boost the Human Growth Hormone (HGH) -

The human growth hormone is secreted by the pituitary gland, which controls a lot of master functions within the body. Some of its main responsibilities have to do with maintaining, building, and repairing healthy tissues in the brain and other organs. Higher levels of this human growth hormone lead to an improved immune system, good heart health, and better sleeping patterns. In terms of fasting, studies show that HGH levels are highest first thing in the morning because your body has been in a fasted state overnight, but as soon as you eat, those levels start to drop. By fasting on a regular basis, you can extend the life of HGH secretion and reap more benefits.

Increase Energy -

Digesting food all throughout the day can be very tiresome for your body, which makes fasting a great method to give your digestive system a little break. When your body is no longer forced to digest food during every waking moment, it can spend more time healing and repairing old or damaged cells, as well as resting and recovering in general. As a result, both your body and your mind will have a chance to unwind from your otherwise hectic schedule, leaving you feeling more energized for the tasks ahead. Furthermore, once your body learns that it should turn to fat for fuel rather than glucose, you will find that your energy is more consistent throughout the day. This is because tapping into fat reserves for fuel means the energy crashes caused by drops in insulin won't occur.

Improve Brain Function -

When the body recognizes that it is fasting, the brain goes into somewhat of a survival mode and becomes hyper-focused in order to preserve whatever stored energy it has for the task at hand. This means that the mind is less likely to wander, resulting in increased efficiency and productivity during the workday. Animal research also suggests that intermittent fasting may suppress inflammation in the brain and lead to better learning and memory. Since brain inflammation is linked to a number of neurological conditions such as Alzheimer's disease, Parkinson's disease, and stroke, suppressing such inflammation may reduce the risk of these neurological disorders.

Help Treat Depression -

It appears that focus isn't the only brain benefit which could result from intermittent fasting, in fact, your mood may improve as well. Two physiological factors called brain-derived neurotrophic factor and ghrelin are at play here, and fasting can raise the levels of both. The brain-derived neurotrophic factor is important for the proper functioning of neuronal networks while ghrelin, also known as the hunger hormone, promotes neurogenesis and is associated with both an elevated mood and overall mood control. Depressed patients have low levels of both BDNF and ghrelin, so increasing these levels by fasting may be helpful in the treatment of depression.

Reduce the Risk of Cancer -
While the research on cancer and intermittent fasting has mostly focused on animals thus far, there are reasons to believe that fasting can help reduce the risk of cancer. For one, since obesity is a risk factor in many different cancers and fasting often leads to weight loss, adopting this eating pattern may help reduce this particular risk factor. Next, decreasing some of the biological factors linked to cancer, such as insulin levels and inflammation, may lower your overall risk. Lastly, since cancer is characterized by uncontrolled cell growth, the beneficial effect that fasting can have on metabolism may lead to a reduction in the risk of cancer. On a slightly different note, there is also some evidence to support that fasting can reduce the side effects of chemotherapy for patients who are currently undergoing cancer treatment.

Promote Longevity -

If the apparent benefits of intermittent fasting hold true, it should come as no surprise that this way of eating may actually help you live longer. Between reducing the risk of diseases such as diabetes and cancer, treating mental illness such as depression, improving brain function such as learning and memory, and more, there are many reasons to believe that intermittent fasting is the key to a healthy and happy life.

Another factor known to affect longevity and aging is the mitochondria, popularly known as the powerhouse of the cell, and fasting may make this powerhouse even stronger. One result that we have seen from fasting is that the cells in your body become more resilient. Resilient cells help hold mitochondrial networks together which keeps the mitochondria strong, thereby processing energy more efficiently and promoting longevity.

*Common Concerns*

While the health benefits associated with fasting look and sound promising, this type of eating schedule is not necessarily a good fit for everyone. Individuals suffering from conditions such as diabetes or low blood sugar should be very cautious, as fasting can lead to spikes and crashes of blood sugar levels. Individuals who are underweight or have previously struggled with disordered eating should consult their doctor before attempting any sort of dietary restriction program. Adolescents, older adults, and pregnant women should be extra mindful of the risks involved with fasting, since their bodies may be in a more delicate state and require greater care. And these are just some of the at-risk categories. Aside from this, there are also some general concerns which anyone thinking about intermittent fasting should consider.

Limited Research -

> Intermittent fasting is still a relatively new concept and while there are constantly new studies coming out with supporting research, much about this lifestyle remains unknown. Most of the studies on fasting thus far have either been carried out on animals or with a small sample of humans, and often with very few trials. Researchers also have no way to assess the long-term effects of fasting since it has only really been around for a decade. This means that there is no knowledge of what problems may arise down the road, or which dangers may present themselves later on.

Not Sustainable -

> For many individuals, their lives do not revolve around food and fitness. While intermittent fasting may be sustainable in the short run, research

suggests that it most likely won't last in the long run. Between inconsistent sleep schedules, varying working days, family dinners, traveling, and events such as weddings and birthdays, intermittent fasting may become difficult to stick to. In fact, the dropout rate for fasters is much higher than that of calorie-cutters. This is why it's important for people getting started with intermittent fasting to think of it as a lifestyle, rather than a form of crash dieting.

Disordered Eating -

Following any sort of eating regimen can lead to an unhealthy obsession with food or a disordered mentality around eating, which may lead to bigger problems down the road. It's not uncommon for intermittent fasters to swap between a highly restrictive mindset while fasting and an all-out binging mindset while eating, even though intermittent fasting does not promote these mindsets. Eating disorders affect individuals of all ages and genders, and while skipping a meal or two may seem harmless, it can quickly become dangerous. Needless to say, those with a history of anorexia nervosa, bulimia nervosa, binge eating disorder, or any other eating disorder should not attempt this lifestyle.

Infertility -

The restrictive nature of intermittent fasting may interfere with the fertility of women due to the stress it can have on the body's reproductive system. The female body is very delicate and when it believes that it is not receiving an adequate number of calories or nutrients to potentially support a baby, it may stop producing eggs and shut down its reproductive system. This can lead to hormonal imbalances and a change in menstrual patterns. One of these changes may be amenorrhea, a term used to refer to the absence of menstruation, which may result in infertility.

Food Sensitivities -

After a period of fasting, you may find it more difficult to say no to cravings. If you choose to give in to these cravings during your eating window and indulge in greasy junk food, you may create a leaky gut. The more scientific name for a leaky gut is intestinal permeability, a condition in which the lining of the small intestine becomes damaged and allows bacteria and toxins to pass into the bloodstream. This can result in food intolerances, inflammation, weight loss resistance, and other gut issues such as gas and bloating. A common gut issue is known by the name of small intestinal bacterial overgrowth, or SIBO, and occurs when excessive bacteria has found its way into your small intestine. This can lead to a variety of food sensitivities, the most common being foods which contain sugar, dairy, or gluten.

Athletic Performance -

Food is fuel, and training in a fasted state can hinder your performance both in and out of the gym. When your carbohydrate stores become depleted, as they do while fasting, the body will turn to fat and protein for energy. Although advocates of fasting claim that the body will use its fat reserves before it breaks down its muscle, others believe that this way of eating may have negative effects on muscle mass and metabolism. Simply put, further research is still needed to understand if the human body burns muscle in addition to fat when its preferred carbohydrate energy source isn't available. What we do know is that training in a fasted state does not provide the same strength and energy as training in a fed state does, thereby hindering athletic performance.

Cortisol Problems -

Cortisol is known as the stress hormone, and it plays a large role in the body's ability to respond to stress. Practicing intermittent fasting for any period of time can lead to elevated levels of this stress hormone, and long-term fasting may lead to problems of chronically elevated cortisol. Since fasting is a form of stress on the body, your systems may not know how to handle the added stress which may produce undesirable effects. Women, in particular, have been known to store extra fat and possibly break down muscle due to the increase in cortisol. That said, exercise is a form of stress on the body in the same way that fasting is, so stress in and of itself is not necessarily a bad thing.

Anxiety -

An increase in the stress hormone cortisol, as mentioned above, can lead to higher levels of anxiety just as it does stress, but this isn't the only way that fasting and anxiety are related. Many intermittent fasters will rely heavily on caffeine during their fasting hours, and this makes it very easy to overdo the amount of coffee or other caffeinated drinks that they consume. Just as hunger can increase cortisol, the jittery effects of caffeine increase levels of anxiety. Higher levels of anxiety can then translate into depression and insomnia.

Sleep Issues -

The most widespread intermittent fasting schedules involve consuming a high number of calories within a couple hours of bedtime. Having such a large meal immediately before going to bed can leave you feeling wide awake, especially if this meal is high in refined carbohydrates. The reason for this goes back to the relationship between carbohydrates and blood sugar. When you eat a high-carb meal right before bed, your blood sugar will crash at various time throughout the night, and this can disrupt your sleep. Therefore, it is therefore best to either stop eating a few hours prior to bedtime, or at least limit the number of carbohydrates at night, focusing mainly on fats and protein instead.

*Possible Side Effects*

In addition to the long list of concerns that go hand in hand with the intermittent fasting lifestyle, there are a number of side effects to be aware of. The good news is that these symptoms are usually short-lived and are not a cause for concern. With that said, always listen to your body and use your best judgment to decide whether it may be time to quit. Intermittent fasting should complement your lifestyle, not complicate it. If any of these symptoms last for more than one week, you may want to consult a doctor or take a break from fasting all together to see if the side effects subside.

Hunger -

As with any changes to eating habits, your body will need some time to adjust. During this so-called adjustment period, hunger is to be expected since research shows we tend to get hungry when we are used to eating. In this respect, intermittent fasting can actually be a handy tool in learning how to differentiate between physical hunger and mental hunger. The longer that you maintain this new eating pattern, the easier it will be to understand and control your different types of hunger. Furthermore, studies claim that regular fasting may actually have an appetite blunting effect, so once your body has fully adjusted to this new eating pattern, you should feel more satiated throughout the day.

Cravings -

In addition to craving food in general, you may find that you crave certain types of foods. The reasoning behind this is similar to the reasoning behind hunger. If you are used to eating the same thing at the same time every single day, it's not uncommon to crave this specific food or meal. A separate type of craving you may have, independent of your prior dietary habits, is for sugar. The preferred source of energy for your body is carbohydrates, and when you begin depleting this energy source as you transition into the fasting lifestyle, you may start to crave sugar while your body figures out where to get its fuel from now. Once your body learns to tap into its fat reserves and use this for fuel instead, intermittent fasting can actually help to reduce your sugar cravings.

Irritability and Low Energy -

It's quite common to feel irritable and deprived of energy while fasting, especially in the beginning. This could be due to a number of things including low blood sugar and sugar withdrawal. If your diet previously consisted of refined sugar and corn syrup, suddenly removing these foods can make you feel cranky and annoyed.

You could also be experiencing irritability and low energy as a result of always having to fight off hunger, cravings, and other side effects. As for feelings of sluggishness and sleepiness, your body is probably just adjusting to using fat for energy. However, this should pass in due time.

Headaches -

There are several reasons that you could be experiencing headaches as a result of intermittent fasting. For one, fasting blood sugar levels sometimes fall too low, which can lead to headaches. Two, since fasting is a form of stress on the body, elevated cortisol levels could be to blame. Third, if you are having trouble sleeping due to eating too close to bedtime or drinking too much caffeine, your restlessness at night could be causing your headaches during the day. Fourth, dehydration could be the culprit. Since you are not receiving as much hydration from foods while fasting, you need to be drinking more water than you may be used to.

Constipation and Heartburn -

When you suddenly introduce an unfamiliar eating pattern to your body, you may experience irregular bowel movements and heartburn. Constipation typically leads to bloating while heartburn typically leads to burping, both of which may be accompanied by mild discomfort or full on pain. Reasons for constipation include dehydration and infrequent meals, while heartburn is due to acid regurgitation. When you don't use the acid produced by your stomach to digest food, this acid backs up into your throat and creates that unpleasant sour taste in your mouth.

These are just some of the common side effects that those who are new to fasting may experience during their transition into the lifestyle. A few things which might help alleviate these symptoms include willpower to fight hunger and cravings, drinking lots of water to prevent dehydration, keeping busy to keep your mind off food, going easy on your workouts to reduce stress, prioritizing sleep to ensure that you are well rested, and incorporating some form of yoga or meditation to help you relax.

# Chapter Three - Intermittent Fasting and Veganism

*Similarities*

When you look at the fundamental principles of intermittent fasting and the fundamental principles of veganism, you may find that these two lifestyles actually share quite a bit in common. While intermittent fasting acts as a guideline for *when* you can eat and veganism lays down a framework for *what* you can eat, how you choose to incorporate each of these principles into your life really comes down to personal preference. Both intermittent fasters and vegans often come from a place of caring for their health and wanting to do what is best for their bodies, and these desires are reflected in the shared principles between these two lifestyles.

Lifestyle, Not a Diet -

> We hear it all the time - *this is a lifestyle, not a diet* - but in the case of both intermittent fasting and veganism, it really is the truth. A diet will often come with a grocery list, a meal plan, a set of instructions, and an overall restrictive approach to eating. Lifestyles, on the other hand, are flexible and focus instead on the ways in which this new way of eating can work for you. Intermittent

fasting and veganism simply provide frameworks to guide you down the right path, but they still leave plenty of room to play around with the variations and find what method will suit your current lifestyle best.

Various Beliefs -

With these being lifestyles rather than diets, both intermittent fasting and veganism are built on some pretty deep-rooted beliefs, but these beliefs often vary from one person to the next. Those who are strong supporters of intermittent fasting may believe in the physical health benefits, the mental health benefits, or the religious and spiritual reasons. Those who stand behind veganism may do it for the animals, the environment, or their own well-being. What makes both intermittent fasting and veganism so widespread is the fact that they are flexible and all-encompassing. No matter what you believe in at your core, certain aspects of these lifestyles can and will resonate with you to some degree.

Importance of Exercise -

As with any healthy lifestyle, engaging in some form of physical activity on a regular basis is just as important as eating a well-balanced diet. Being conscious of what you are putting into your body often goes hand in hand with paying attention to how you are moving your body, and that is indeed the case with these lifestyles. Sure, the intermittent fasting community may lean more toward weight lifting and extreme sports while the vegan community may promote yoga and long-distance running, but these are of course just stereotypes and generalizations. At the end of the day, exercise is exercise, and both fasting and veganism promote an all-around healthy lifestyle, inclusive of both physical and mental health.

Food Quality -

Whether you're a hard-core faster or a hard-core vegan, chances are you probably care about the types of foods that you are putting in your body. What makes these lifestyles realistic and sustainable for most people is that they preach eating whole, nutrient-dense foods and staying away from processed junk. The recommended breakdown of protein, carbohydrates, and fats may differ from one source to the next, but a diet consisting of mainly natural, high-quality foods is something that everyone can agree on. This can then lead to greater nutritional awareness and may even help eliminate nutrient deficiencies.

Disease Prevention -

The body's ability to prevent and overcome various diseases through diet and exercise is truly astonishing. The fact that both intermittent fasting and veganism encourage and promote a balanced lifestyle consisting of healthy disease-fighting foods and regular physical activity makes them both conducive to disease prevention. On one hand, intermittent fasting claims to reduce the risk of cancer and various neurological disorders, while on the other hand, veganism claims to be the best approach for the prevention of heart disease and other chronic diseases. The approaches of these lifestyles and the types of diseases they benefit may differ, but their focus on health promotion is undoubtedly the same across the board.

## Differences

The fundamental principles of intermittent fasting and veganism certainly overlap to some degree, but a few obvious differences exist as well. In some cases, these differences are minor and perhaps insignificant, but there are specific issues in which these lifestyles seem to stand at polar opposites. Despite these apparent contradictions at times, there are ways to make such dissimilarities work for you and your lifestyle. After all, the appeal of both intermittent fasting and veganism lies in the flexibility that these ways of eating allow.

Dietary Conditions -

Intermittent fasting was first popularized by muscular men in the fitness industry who were basically living on chicken breasts, raw egg whites, and whey protein shakes. Veganism, on the other hand, was built on the belief that humans should not consume any foods that come from animal sources in order to prevent the exploitation of these beings. Over the years, this concern for animals has extended to include the health and environmental benefits of a plant-based diet as well. The main difference in dietary conditions between these two lifestyles comes about in the discussion of protein, specifically the effect of animal protein versus plant protein. Many people in the intermittent fasting community believe that a high-protein diet consisting mainly of animal products will give the best results, while the vegan community as a whole advocate for a diet rich in plant protein, healthy fats, and complex carbohydrates. As such, you'll sometimes hear people say that you can be a vegan intermittent faster, but you can't be an intermittent fasting vegan.

Carbohydrate Intake -

Taking the discussion of dietary conditions one step further, the topic of carbohydrates is of particular importance in the worlds of intermittent fasting and veganism. Eating a high-carb diet while intermittent fasting can be counterproductive due to the relationship between carbohydrates and blood sugar. When you ingest carbohydrates, your body breaks it down into sugar and your blood sugar levels rise, increasing your insulin levels. As we know, an increase in insulin can lead to undesirable weight gain. A vegan diet, however, is naturally fairly high in carbohydrates, and this can be difficult to avoid. Even if you eat a high-protein, high-fat vegan diet, plant-based protein sources such as quinoa, chickpeas, lentils, Ezekiel bread, and vegetables don't come without some added carbohydrates too.

Availability of Information -

The term intermittent fasting has only been around since 2006 while the term vegan was coined back in 1944, making veganism a much more researched and scientifically advanced practice. Opinions are of course always changing, especially with the diet mentality that continues to plague our society today, but the vegan diet is certainly more understood regarding long-term benefits and potential risks. There are even individuals on this earth who have been fully vegan for life. Apart from the research side things, there are also just more sources out there to learn about the vegan diet in general. From cookbooks and blog posts to podcasts and personal experience, the information that is available to the public makes it easier for potential vegans to make an educated and informed decision.

*The Compound Benefits*

Intermittent fasting and veganism each provide tremendous results on their own and when combined, the benefits of these two lifestyles fuse together effortlessly. The combination of intermittent fasting and a whole food plant-based diet can actually reduce your risk of disease more than either approach ever could on its own, partly because combining the teachings of these two methods results in a highly anti-inflammatory way of eating. And this is just one of the many ways that incorporating intermittent fasting into your vegan lifestyle can be beneficial.

Reduced Inflammation -

People typically experience inflammation when the body is trying to heal itself. This means that inflammation in and of itself is not a bad thing, but when your insides are inflamed for extended periods of time, it can lead to some very negative health outcomes. Both intermittent fasting and veganism significantly reduce inflammation in the body due to calorie restriction and dietary fiber, respectively. Calorie restriction leads to autophagy, ketogenesis, and insulin sensitivity, all of which reduce inflammation. Similarly, a diet rich in fiber will reduce inflammation, possibly due to plant chemicals called phytonutrients found in fiber-rich fruits and vegetables. Additional anti-inflammatory vegan foods include leafy greens, sweet potatoes, blueberries, nuts and seeds, soy products, whole grains, turmeric, and garlic.

Weight Loss -

Individuals turn to intermittent fasting and veganism for a variety of reasons, and weight loss is often number one. This is actually quite interesting because neither of these lifestyles primarily market themselves to the weight loss community, but people are intrigued by the results that they see in other people. When it comes down to it, weight loss is a simple equation of calories in versus calories out, and intermittent fasting and veganism make it easier to maintain a calorie deficit. By limiting the time in which you eat to an 8-hour eating window and consuming a diet built around whole, plant-based foods, people naturally tend to consume fewer calories and lose weight.

Simplified Lifestyle -

Intermittent fasting and veganism may sound complicated enough on their own, but combining these lifestyles can actually simplify your life more than you think. The fasting schedule will conveniently dictate *when* you eat and the vegan diet will lay out *what* you eat at those pre-planned meal times, making the rest fall into place almost effortlessly. Human nature has a way of overcomplicating even the simplest of things, so don't let your diet and lifestyle be the victim of this tendency. Sure, it may take a few weeks of trial and error to figure out what works best for you, but it won't be long before you start reaping some significant benefits.

*The Compound Concerns*

Just as intermittent fasting and veganism provide tremendous benefits both on their own and together, they also raise some concerns. A lifestyle which includes both fasting and a vegan diet means that you have to take extra precautions to ensure that you are getting enough macronutrients and micronutrients from the foods you are eating. It also means that you now not only need to think about the foods which you are consuming, but also the times in which you are consuming them. This may feel somewhat like a puzzle at the start, but with a little bit of experimentation, the pieces should fit together soon enough.

Digestive Problems -

Any change in diet or lifestyle, no matter how big or small, can lead to a number of digestion issues. Even if you are implementing intermittent fasting on an already vegan diet, you may still experience symptoms such as constipation, diarrhea, and bloating. Since the bacteria in your gut is optimized for the types of foods you normally eat, a simple shift such as going from high-carb, low-fat to high-fat, high-protein could wreak havoc on your digestive system. By changing your eating patterns slowly over time, you may be able to alleviate some of this digestive distress.

Social Limitations -

Being vegan in a meat-eating world can be difficult enough as it is, especially when it comes to social situations. Add intermittent fasting on top of that, and you now have a whole other factor in the equation that you need to solve. Say that you're making brunch plans with friends, as an example. You're probably used to checking the menu for vegan options, but now you also need to agree on a time that fits within your eating window. Then of course there are those individuals who just don't understand why you lead the lifestyle that you do, which can result in them mocking and ridiculing you. These two things combined can be both frustrating and exhausting, making social situations a cause of stress rather than a form of enjoyment.

Overall Health -

Following a vegan diet means that you need to be extra mindful of the things you are putting into your body to ensure that you are not deficient in any nutrients or vitamins. For example, most doctors agree that all vegans should be supplementing B12 since it's just not possible to fulfill this need on a plant-based diet. Being deficient in vitamins and minerals can lead to things such as bad skin, brittle hair and nails, low energy, muscle cramps, brain fog, and poor sleep. Since many of these symptoms are the same ones that can occur in connection with intermittent fasting, you want to be careful not to worsen the effects.

# Chapter Four - How to Implement Intermittent Fasting

*Getting Started*

The health benefits of intermittent fasting alone plus the compound benefits that result when intermittent fasting is introduced into a vegan diet are difficult to ignore. The good news is, implementing this new pattern of eating can really be quite simple in practice, given that you stick to the general guidelines and follow the most important rules. These are mostly concerned with how to properly start and break a fast, as well as what you should and shouldn't do during a fasting period.

Recommended Method -

The 16:8 Method is the one that is recommended for beginners because it is easy to implement and helps ease the transition into fasting. Since the average person naturally fasts for 8 to 12 hours overnight, extending this fasting period to 16 hours usually just means skipping breakfast. Once you break your fast around midday, you then have 8 hours to consume your daily calories, macronutrients, and micronutrients. This is just about as basic as intermittent fasting gets, but there are some additional considerations to be made. The foods you consume immediately prior to and after a fast can have a massive impact on how your body responds to intermittent fasting, so it's important to get it right.

Starting a Fast -

Before you begin a fast, it is best to consume a meal that is high in fiber because this will put you in a situation where you are a little more satiated. The vegan diet is typically fairly high in fiber to begin with, but it wouldn't hurt to add some extra vegetables or a couple teaspoons of psyllium husk. Eating these fiber-rich foods immediately before a fast will still give you all the metabolic benefits of fasting without the drawbacks such as a grumbling stomach and other feelings of hunger. A small amount of fats, such as coconut oil, is also helpful because although fats take a bit longer to digest, the fatty acids that they leak into the bloodstream will help your liver produce ketone bodies.

Breaking a Fast -

When breaking a fast, it is best not to consume fats with carbohydrates. This is because carbohydrates cause an insulin spike and this makes cells receptive of whatever was just consumed, so in this case, both the carbohydrates and the fats will find their way into the cells.

On the other hand, if you just consume carbs by themselves, only carbs will go into the cells and if you just consume fats, they won't trigger an insulin response at all so the cell won't even open. In sum, consume carbohydrates with protein or fats with protein immediately following a period of fasting. Some foods which are high-carb, high-protein, low-fat include quinoa, oats, nutritional yeast, spinach, and legumes, while those that are high-fat, high-protein, and relatively low-carb include nut butters, chia seeds, and tofu.

Liquids -

With the exception of dry fasting, a type of fast in which you do not consume any liquids, drinking beverages with zero calories is allowed and encouraged during a period of fasting. This includes water, black coffee, and tea, although it is extremely important that you don't add any sweeteners or creamers as this can trigger an insulin response. Some studies actually suggest that black coffee may support your fast because the polyphenols in both caffeinated and decaffeinated coffee encourage cells to undergo autophagy, thereby speeding up the process of cell recycling. If weight loss is your goal, drinking black coffee may help with this as well because caffeine is proven to speed up your metabolism.

Alcohol -

One liquid which is often up for debate, both within the intermittent fasting community and outside thereof, is alcohol. When it comes to fasting, it is recommended that you only drink alcohol during your eating window for obvious reasons. Since drinking on an empty stomach will cause the alcohol to be absorbed directly into the bloodstream through the stomach, you will feel drunker in a shorter period of time. Therefore, if you do decide to drink, make sure to do so on a full stomach and drink a lot of water. Of course, consuming alcohol will have no benefit on your health or fitness goals, so it is best that you do it in moderation.

Exercise -

The topic of exercise in connection with intermittent fasting is widely discussed, both within the fitness community and across the general public. When it comes down to it, whether you exercise while fasted or fed really just comes down to personal preference. Sure, some people advocate for exercising on an empty stomach immediately prior to breaking your fast, and then there are others who believe exercising at the end of your eating window is far more beneficial because this is the only time you have adequate energy to push yourself. Both of these arguments are completely valid, so pick the time that fits with your schedule and works best for you. The most important thing is that you get your body moving since any exercise is better than no exercise at all.

*Beginner Mistakes*

Given all the things to consider when embarking on an intermittent fasting journey for the first time, you will most likely make some mistakes along the way. In order to achieve the maximum benefits from this pattern of eating, it's important that you follow the rules and guidelines above to the best of your ability. Living according to these parameters will feel effortless in due time, but it can definitely be a bit tricky and slightly frustrating at the start, hence this list of beginner mistakes. Becoming aware of these common stumbling blocks and pitfalls will make you better equipped to bypass them in your transition, increasing your chances of success with this new lifestyle.

Giving Up Too Soon -

> The adjustment period into an intermittent fasting lifestyle can last anywhere from a week to a month, and this can make people throw in the towel much too soon. As discussed previously, side effects such as hunger and cravings, constipation and

heartburn, irritability and low energy, and headaches are fairly common, so wanting to quit is understandable. The benefits, however, lie on the other side of this roadblock, so it's important to continue pushing and get over this hurdle. You probably encountered some similar side effects when first transitioning to a plant-based diet, so use this knowledge as a source of encouragement and remind yourself that the side effects will pass.

Forgetting Your Why -

Chances are that you felt drawn to intermittent fasting for a reason, perhaps you want to lose weight and tone up, or maybe you just see this as a challenge to become mentally and physically stronger. Whatever the reason may be, zero in on accomplishing what you set out to do in the first place and don't lose sight of your goals. This can also help with the mistake of giving up too soon, as mentioned above. The dropout rate for fasters is already extremely high, so don't just become another statistic.

Drinking Too Little Water -

The last thing you want to do during a fast is put added stress on your body. When you are in a fasted state, your body begins to detox itself and break down damaged components. During this process, water is essential in order to flush out the toxins properly. Going for long periods of time without ingesting any food can also dehydrate your cells. Since you are not consuming any hydrating foods such as fruits and vegetables, all your hydration needs now must come in the form of liquids. Drinking more water will also make you feel full and decrease feelings of hunger, easing the transition into fasting as well.

Eating the Wrong Foods -

The stomach has something called dispensability which means that it will shrink as a result of regular fasting intervals. If you are not deliberate in the way that you structure your meals, it's far too easy to fill up on non-nutritious foods, leaving no room in your stomach for the fresh ingredients and nutrients that your body needs to function properly. On a similar note, some people will use intermittent fasting as an excuse to indulge in anything they please, which is something to be extra cautious of. This method of eating is by no means a magic fix and at the end of the day, the simple equation of calories in versus calories out will determine whether you gain or lose weight with this lifestyle.

Not Eating Enough -

Just because intermittent fasting promotes skipping meals doesn't mean you're supposed to drastically cut your calories, or reduce your intake at all, for that matter. Your body needs energy to function, and calories are merely a form of energy. When you don't eat enough, you may experience low energy and find that you are always thinking about food or constantly feeling cold. These are all signs that your body isn't receiving the minimum number of calories it needs to function. Not eating enough for extended periods of time can eventually lead to binge eating and other forms of disordered eating in the future, so you want to make sure that you are fueling your body properly from the start.

Eating Too Much -

It's sometimes difficult to find the right balance between eating too little and eating too much during your eating window, and overeating can be just as dangerous as undereating. Reasons that you may overindulge, whether it is intentional or not, include feeling famished, believing that you can eat whatever you want, and thinking that you need to stuff yourself now so that you won't be hungry later. Snacking all throughout your eating window is also a huge mistake because each time you ingest even the smallest number of calories, your insulin levels will spike. This spike in insulin prevents fat burning and encourages this fat to be stored instead, which is exactly what you don't want.

Choosing the Wrong Method -

>With so many different types of fasting out there, it's crucial to find the one that suits you and your lifestyle best. While the 16:8 Method comes highly recommended for beginners, that doesn't mean it's the one you need to go with. People have different jobs, schedules, home lives, and so on, so you're better off choosing the plan that will be easiest to maintain. Intermittent fasting is all about trial and error so if you start with one method and decide to switch to another one, that is perfectly fine.

Going to Extremes -

>The reason that diet dropout rates are so high is that people take an all or nothing approach and end up going to extremes. Dedication and consistency are key, but don't let these things get in the way of the bigger picture. Your approach to intermittent fasting should be both realistic and sustainable, so remember to treat yourself every once in a while. Eat not only for physical health, but also for your mental health and your soul.

*Common Myths*

Before summarizing the fundamental principles of intermittent fasting, it may be helpful to address and debunk some of the most common myths associated with the lifestyle. Given the amount of media attention that intermittent fasting has received in recent years, there have been a significant number of critics and skeptics who have had quite a bit to say on the topic. Now that a lot of these myths are finally being put to rest due to new evidence and continued research, it's time to debunk some of the most popular beliefs surrounding the intermittent fasting lifestyle.

Myth: Intermittent fasting will slow down your metabolism.

> This is probably the one you hear most often, and it's for a good reason. In the mid-1900s, it was believed that you should eat three medium-sized meals per day. In the early-2000s, this then jumped to eating six small meals every 2 to 3 hours, claiming that this would boost your metabolism and help you burn more calories throughout the day. Intermittent fasting of course goes against this belief, but there is research to suggest that your metabolic rate may actually benefit from periods of fasting, as long as you are not restricting your calories. When you fast for 16 hours or more, you release a hormone called norepinephrine. This hormone functions as both a stress hormone and a neurotransmitter, and recent studies suggest that the release of this hormone can actually increase your resting metabolic rate.

Myth: Intermittent fasting can put your body in starvation mode.

Starvation mode is a term that is often thrown around in both the fasting community and the dieting industry, but starvation is in no way the same thing as fasting or dieting. In short, starvation mode refers to a situation in which your body believes it is starving, therefore shutting down its metabolism and preventing your body from burning fat. The more technical term for this is adaptive thermogenesis and it is a real thing, but not in the context that people use it. There is no evidence to suggest that cycling between periods of fasting and periods of eating will make your body believe that it is starving. As stated above, fasts greater than 16 hours can actually increase your metabolism.

Myth: Intermittent fasting will lead to muscle loss.

Critics of intermittent fasting like to say that our bodies will use muscle as fuel instead of fat, but that makes no sense when there is still an abundance of fat to burn. The evolutionary reason that humans store fat on their bodies is so that they have a backup source of energy when food is not available. Tapping into fat reserves is therefore a very natural process during a fast, which is how intermittent fasting really came to be in the first place. That's not to say that no muscle will be lost in the process, but you will certainly lose far more fat than you will muscle.

Myth: Intermittent fasting is not for women.
Some people fear that implementing intermittent fasting as a woman is not safe due to the added complexities of hormones and reproductive systems. While it is definitely true that females are more sensitive to hunger hormones and will need to take extra precautions when it comes to their reproductive health, intermittent fasting is perfectly safe for women. The reason that females may experience a change in their menstrual pattern, such as longer or less regular cycles, is because the body doesn't know when it will be fed next. While your body learns to trust this new eating pattern, it may stop producing eggs as to not stimulate its reproductive system. This is simply a defense mechanism which will most likely subside once intermittent fasting becomes the new norm.

Myth: Intermittent fasting will stunt your growth.
There is some debate around whether or not children and adolescents should intermittent fast due to the concern that it may stunt their growth. This concern stems from the belief that prolonged periods of fasting will deprive your body of the nutrients it needs to grow. The fact of the matter is

any diet that is lacking in adequate macronutrients and micronutrients may stunt your growth, but fasting alone is not the culprit. That said, if you find that fasting makes it more difficult to reach your nutrition goals, it may not be the right choice at this time in your life.

Myth: Intermittent fasting is detrimental to your health. Without knowing the mechanisms at play, it's understandable why some people may view calorie restriction and regular fasting as harmful, but this really couldn't be further from the truth. The benefits of intermittent fasting are plenty, such as improved insulin sensitivity, reduced inflammation, enhanced brain function, and a decreased risk of cancer, diabetes, heart disease, and other diseases. As with any type of eating regimen, you still need to make sure that you are eating a well-balanced diet rich in micronutrients, but intermittent fasting in and of itself is by no means terrible for your health.

# Chapter Five - Intermittent Fasting Summary

*Conclusion*

At the very core, intermittent fasting is an eating pattern that is built around periods of fasting and windows of eating. By redirecting the focus from *what* you consume to *when* you consume it, this way of eating presents itself as a lifestyle rather than a diet. The flexibility regarding how you fast, when you fast, and what you eat during a fast makes intermittent fasting suitable for a variety of lifestyles and dietary restrictions. As long as you follow the general guidelines and fundamental principles of fasting, there's really no wrong way to go about it.

The intention behind intermittent fasting is to cycle your body between a fasted state and a fed state in order to reap a variety of health benefits. These benefits may be even greater when combined with a vegan diet and range from weight loss and improved brain function to reduced inflammation and prevention of disease. On the downside, there are a number of concerns that come along with this type of fasting as well. These concerns range from disordered eating and food sensitivities to cortisol problems and infertility. Depending on your health background and prior dietary regimen, you may be at a greater risk for experiencing some of these downsides.

While much about the intermittent fasting lifestyle has yet to be understood from a scientific standpoint, especially as it relates to veganism, the results that people have experienced are overall favorable. As with any diet regimen, it's important to do your research and determine if intermittent fasting is right for you. It may also be beneficial to consult a professional or get a second opinion from someone you trust. At the end of the day, you are responsible for your body, and how you decide to treat it is completely up to you.

www.ingramcontent.com/pod-product-compliance
Lightning Source LLC
Chambersburg PA
CBHW071238240726
48654CB00009B/1097